M000190374

Salt

Explore the Dark Side of the All-American Meal, America's Food Addiction, and Why We Get Fat by Understanding How the Food Giants Hooked Us On Mindless Eating

Alexandra Kastor

Salt Sugar Fat

Explore the Dark Side of the All-American Meal, America's Food Addiction, and Why We Get Fat by Understanding How the Food Giants Hooked Us On Mindless Eating

© Copyright 2013 Alexandra Kastor & affiliates

Reproduction or translation of any part of this work beyond that permitted by section 107 or 108 of the 1976 United States Copyright Act without permission of the copyright owner is unlawful. Requests for permission or further information should be addressed to the author.

This publication is designed to provide accurate and authoritative information in regard to the subject matter covered. It is sold with the understanding that the publisher, author, and affiliates are not engaged in rendering legal, accounting, or any other professional services. This includes medical advice. The author of this book is not a doctor and does not claim to be one. If legal advice or other expert assistance is required, the services of a competent professional person should be sought.

ISBN-13: **978-0615880730**
ISBN-10: **0615880738**

First Published, 2013
United States of America

Special Thanks to You!

As a special thanks to you, our reader, please accept this FREE gift!

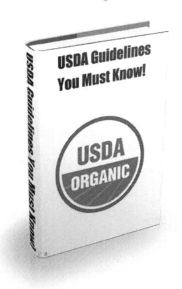

Purchasing this book may have been the first step of your journey to a better life. As a thank you for your purchase, and to help you on this journey, I would like to provide to you a **USDA Organic Guidelines Report Absolutely FREE.**
Download at:
alexandsteven.com/signups/saltsugarfat

TABLE OF CONTENTS

DEDICATION

This book is dedicated to one of the biggest inspirations in my life:

My Mom, Kathleen Kastor.

You have lead me on a path to a healthy life from the time I was young, I am lucky to have been blessed to be your daughter. I don't know where I would be today without you.

I love you, mom.

Thank you for all you do every day. I couldn't be happier.

-Alex

The American Way

The United States of America, land of the free, home of the brave, birthplace of democracy... and the Big Mac. There are many things the United States of America is known for, but above all I'd say right now our waistlines hold the most weight. We live in a media driven society; a country full of advertisements and force-fed manipulation.

Now, advertisements aren't inherently bad, but the manipulative tactics utilized on the ill-informed American public are.

Although studies have been performed which prove the vast majority of the population does not have much confidence in the media, I don't believe Americans take enough action in response to their lack of faith in it.

According to an article by marketplace.org, processed foods make up approximately 70 percent of the US populace's diet. These findings completely contradict the previously stated study because if we didn't trust the media, why would we buy the products they push on television, radio, billboards, in magazines, and on the internet? There's one of two scenarios occurring here; either the majority of the US is completely confident in the media or we just have no idea what we're doing when it comes to food.

I'm much more inclined to believe that ignorance runs amuck in American society and I believe each and every one of us is guilty as charged or has been at some point in our lives.

American ignorance is the culprit to blame for why our diets consist of nearly 70% processed foods. Don't believe me? What was the last piece of food you ate? Did it have a wrapper or come in a box, bag, or can? Read the ingredients, rather, try to pronounce the ingredients. Pick one of the larger words towards the end of the list.

Do you know what it is? I don't mean a general idea of what it probably is and, "It's a preservative," doesn't count. I mean, do you really know what that ingredient is and the effects it has on your body? If you Google it you most likely will come across a list of dangerous side effects and health risks associated with that ingredient.

We Are Hooked on Cheap Instead of Good-to-Eat

I don't want to insult anyone by referring to Americans as ignorant- I include myself in that generality. There are millions of Americans who are not ignorant and know that processed foods are bad for them, but they buy them anyway to save a few dollars at the grocery store. When you go to the grocery store, there is an extensive amount of products on the shelves to choose from.

You see different products and different prices. Some of us have enough to live comfortably and can purchase what we want but others live paycheck to paycheck. It can be hard to swing the extra cash to purchase the healthier, organic foods rather than the processed products littered around us at the store. Before you justify your action of purchasing processed over organic let me ask you a question.

Can you really not afford it? Are you a smoker? Are you a drinker? Are you a shopper? Are you spending more money on things you like to have rather than spending your cash on the things you need to have? If this is the case, you have no excuse to not be purchasing organic foods.

If you're living paycheck to paycheck and still have time for cigarettes, alcohol, and/or unnecessary, extravagant spending you have absolutely no excuse not to be taking care of yourself and your family properly. If you're one of the people who spends on wants and luxuries and chooses cheaper food your health may suffer. People never expect bad things to happen to them. Ask anyone who has ever been injured in a car accident or has been diagnosed with some disease and they'll give you the answer, "I never thought it could happen to me."

Consider my own brother. My brother is not the unhealthiest guy on the planet; he works out daily and is in pretty decent physical shape on the outside. You see, my brother drinks with his friends every weekend almost ritually.

He eats fast food like Dominos and Taco Bell during beer runs with his buddies. He's dedicated to his weight-lifting routine, so he is sure to take an energy supplement before his workout and a protein supplement after his workout.

My brother is the typical 22-year old; he's in his prime and is virtually indestructible. Or so he thinks. Due to my brother's poor choices regarding what he puts in his body, he has been diagnosed with a serious medical condition known as ulcerative colitis. The processed foods, alcohol, and supplements my brother has been eating over the last few years have badly damaged the surfaces of his intestines.

Some days aren't as bad as others and he can party with his friends like he used to, but whenever he does, he pays for it dearly. He now has to take a pill daily that looks fit for a horse and he heads to the hospital every other week for an IV which is supposed to help nurture his intestines back to health. Ulcerative colitis is not an easy fix. In order to heal properly, diet must change. My brother, like so many others, has this to say about his current health situation: "I never thought it would happen to me."

I would never expect someone to consume a 100% organic diet; I can't even find a way to pull that off myself and I've been trying to be healthy with great dedication for quite some time.

However, if you were able to replace 25%, 50%, or 75% of your processed diet with organic, whole foods, think about what good it would bring to you and your family. Your health is the most precious thing you have- more precious than your house, your car, your money, etc.

You must do everything you can to protect it because an ounce of prevention is worth a pound of cure as the saying goes.

By purchasing this book you've put yourself on the path to proper nutrition and better health. Follow the tips, advice, and guidance in this book and you will be headed on your way to keeping yourself and your loved ones safe from poor health.

I've compiled the information in this book to help teach others what I've learned about keeping yourself safe from the dangers of the modern food industry. I hope that it can help you as it has helped me.

What Consumers Don't Know

Melanie Warner, author of the book *Pandora's Lunchbox*, put out one of the most important pieces of information I've ever encountered during my time studying the health industry. Melanie states,

"The FDA doesn't actually know how many additives are going into our food. This is in part because regulations are not only self-regulatory – so the food industry is doing the testing – but it's also voluntary ... The ingredient companies don't actually have to tell the FDA about a new ingredient. If they choose to, they can simply just launch it into the market. The FDA doesn't know about them, and nobody else really knows about them."

-Melanie Warner, author of Pandora's Lunchbox, during an interview by Kai Ryssdal on marketplace.org

What it comes down to then is that not knowing what you're eating isn't even your fault. The people who are in charge of regulating the ingredients used in your food aren't even aware of what the companies producing the food are putting in them, so how could you? You can't. The only way to avoid the chemicals and everything else that is in processed foods is to stay away from the products. But if you don't know what you're trying to avoid, what can you do to avoid it?

Avoiding Garbage at the Grocery Store

Whenever you're walking through the grocery store, understand that much of what you're looking at is processed and not good for your health. If you're going to avoid these foods, you're going to need to know how to identify them and enable yourself to choose wisely. Here are 10 great tips for avoiding "garbage at the grocery store."

1. Check the ingredients label: The simplest thing you can do to steer yourself and your loved ones clear of unhealthy food is by utilizing the ingredients label on the product. A general rule of thumb is this: If there are many ingredients required to produce the product on the ingredients label, put it back. If there are any words you struggle to pronounce or don't know what they are, once again, place that product back on the shelf.

Never assume you know what an ingredient is unless you know for a fact what it is. Did you know that one of the most dangerous food additives, monosodium glutamate (MSG), has over 32 registered names in order to mask its appearance in food? These names range from simple generic terms like "spice," "broth," "gelatin," and "milk powder" to more complex chemical names like "monopotassium glutamate," "calcium caseinate," and "glutamic acid."

For more of MSG's codenames refer to **elephantjournal.com** via the link in the back of the book. Should you decide not to visit that link, check out this excerpt on the dangers of MSG.

"MSG, or monosodium glutamate, got its reputation as a flavor enhancer extracted from seaweeds in China. In the early 1900's, the process was perfected in Japan and became commercially available. In the 1960's, the phrase "Chinese Restaurant Syndrome" was coined by the New England Journal of Medicine. Twenty minutes after eating Chinese food, some sensitive people would experience tingling, numbness, brain fog, chest pressure and pain. In the 1970's, researchers found that pharmaceutical MSG would kill brain cells in a laboratory. Shortly thereafter, they realized that commercially available MSG would have the same effect."

-Dr. John Douillard, DC, ***Sneaky Names for MSG: Check Your Labels.***

2. Don't fall for the "natural ingredients" ploy: If a product on a store shelf is an organic unadulterated food this will be clearly and proudly displayed on the label. Food manufacturers know this and do everything they can to imitate organic food labeling in order to associate their product with a healthy one. This sneaky tactic the food behemoths employ has completely destroyed the use of the phrases "natural" and "all-natural."

If a food states that it is all-natural, don't just take that at face value. Do your due diligence and analyze the rest of the packaging. Look for phrases such as "non-GMO", "Only one ingredient," "no artificial anything!" and "organic" with a USDA organic logo as shown below.

By being on the lookout for these key words you are on the right path for discerning which are healthy foods and which are not-so-healthy choices.

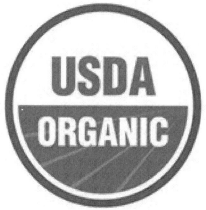

As previously stated, "all-natural" does not mean much. According to the FDA, a company can claim their product is all-natural as long as the food doesn't contain added colors, artificial flavors or "synthetic substances."

This leaves plenty of room for interpretation. If it hasn't become apparent already, this means that a food labeled "natural" can in fact contain preservatives, and often even can contain high fructose corn syrup (which by now we should all know is not a good thing).

3. No sugar/No sugar added: If you're concerned about your calories and carbs due to a condition such as diabetes, you may toss products that indicate a lack of sugar into your shopping cart.

This is a huge mistake and the reason is twofold.

Number one: foods like fruits, milk, many grains, and vegetables all contain natural sugars, so if one of these products is labeled as "no sugar added" you're still looking at a significant amount of sugar intake.

Number two: If a food that you expect to be sweet is labeled as "sugar-free" or "no sugar," run. This product is often loaded with **dangerous chemicals such as aspartame** and **other artificial sweeteners.**

Artificial sweeteners are linked to a host of dangerous side effects including weight gain, depression, seizures, and even cancer. Steer clear of this stuff for lasting health.

4. Zero trans-fat: Chances are, if you're considering a food based on trans-fat content, it isn't healthy. But considering you simply *must* have this product, refer again to the ingredients label. Check for ingredients such as hydrogenated oils. If they're there, the product contains trans-fat and can still claim that there is none (if you ever see hydrogenated oils on an ingredients label, the product is not healthy).

Believe it or not, companies can place 0g of trans-fat on their labels as long as the actual serving contents are *below* 0.5g.

This means that if you use a considerable amount of a "0 trans-fat" product, you could actually be doing a lot of damage to your health. **For the record, trans-fats are directly linked to decreased heart health.**

5. Free range: This is an interesting one. The FDA definition of free range states that the animal in question has been released from its cage and has experienced the outside world; however, it does not state the duration, amount, or quality of outdoor access the animal must achieve.

Basically, as long as a chicken has set foot outside, it can be classified as free range. Instead of looking for free range meats, aim for cage-free, grass-fed, and humanely raised meats. The quality of the meat will be much higher not only in taste and texture, but in nutrition as well.

6. Fat free: Once again, if something that is typically found in a food is missing, it was manipulated in some way to remove it. If your packaging says fat free, it should be something that doesn't ordinarily contain fat because if it does, you're about to purchase a culinary science project. Your body will not thank you for it.

7. **Light and Diet:** Again, if the product you are buying normally has 100 calories and you purchase a "light" version that has 10, those calories were removed by replacing good, natural, healthy ingredients with their chemical counterparts. Do yourself and your body a favor, do not eat 'light' and 'diet' products.

8. **Made with Real…:** Products that boast claims of real fruit or Real® cheese may not contain any actual fruit or ingredients pictured on the box. **One Californian was so enraged by this she actually sued Fruit Roll-Ups because their strawberry fruit roll-up contained no actual strawberries** (Check the back of the book for a link or Google it!). Its flavor was derived from "artificial flavors, sweeteners, and pear juice from concentrate."

Did you notice the capitalized real above with the registered (®) symbol? That's because Kraft macaroni & cheese is made with Real® cheese. Real is actually a company, not an adjective describing their cheese. Sneaky, huh? It's so bad for you, in fact, that it has been scrutinized as being **"basically plastic."**

9. **Organic:** I know what you're thinking, "Alexandra, didn't you just say I should be aiming for organic foods?" Yes, I did.

Tread carefully, though, as manufacturers of processed foods are quite unhappy with the fact that they are losing sales due to their products being thought of as less healthy than organic foods. They are funneling millions upon millions of dollars into the hands of the USDA and FDA in order to manipulate their guidelines for organic foods so that they can get a piece of the action. Organic once meant just that- organic, the word is slowly losing its integrity.

They will try to go down this slippery slope without consumers being aware of the changes. **In order to better understand the USDA guidelines of organic foods visit <u>alexandsteven.com/signups/saltsugarfat</u> and claim a free PDF of the USDA's organic food guidelines.**

10: Table Salt and Sodium: If you're purchasing a product that contains sodium it contains salt. The important concept to note is which type of salt the product contains. If what you're about to buy is not clearly labeled as containing Himalayan salt or sea salt, it probably contains processed table salt. Table salt is a processed version of healthy salt. Processed table salt is not healthy. Salts in nature are not a bleached white color.

They contain trace minerals that are beneficial to your body. Natural salts like Himalayan and sea salts aid in digestion and water retention whereas processed table salts are a factor in hypertension.

Don't fall for the ploy big business throws at you that "you need iodine in your diet" from table salt. This simply is not true. Iodine can be easily obtained from foods such as eggs, and is found in a vast number of foods in trace amounts.

Does this seem like a lot of information? Don't worry; nearly 59% of consumers have a hard time understanding nutrition labels, according to a Nielsen survey.

It's perfectly understandable and although you may feel overwhelmed, don't fret. I'm here to help you understand all of this information because not only do I care about you, your health, and your well-being, but I care about your family's health and well-being also.

When you start with a few labels, before you know it everything starts to make more sense. Just knowing that you need to be checking things more thoroughly puts you ahead of the pack.

Science of Selling: We've Been Fooled!

It is amazing how many people the media can deceive. They continue to tell people what they want to hear and do not care about health in the least. They care about your money and how companies can pocket more of it. Companies know what consumers like and make it addicting. They know that people are busy and have created an industry to satisfy the needs of people on the go, people with low energy and people who are addicted to sugar, salt, additives, and junk food.

If you think about a day in the average person's life, he or she goes to work from about 9 to 5, wakes up early daily, has no energy, and relies on convenient food sources instead of healthy ones. There have been a number of myths about foods that are commonly promoted as "healthy." Dr. Mercola has an article pointing out the **10 most common lies promoted by the "mainstream nutritionists."** I want to give you a brief overview of his 10 reported misconceptions.

The 10 common misconceptions Mercola points out are as follows:

1. 'Saturated Fat Causes Heart Disease.'

Saturated fats that are from animals and different vegetable varieties are what our bodies rely on to function properly. These fats help provide energy and build up our cell membranes and different hormones.

"Saturated fats are also:
- *The preferred fuel for your heart, and also used as a source of fuel during energy expenditure*
- *Useful antiviral agents (caprylic acid)*
- *Effective as an anti-cavity, anti-plaque and anti-fungal agent (lauric acid)*
- *Useful to lower cholesterol levels (palmitic and stearic acids)*
- *Modulators of genetic regulation and prevent cancer (butyric acid)"*

-Dr.Mercola, *10 Lies and Misconceptions Spread By Mainstream Nutrition*

2. 'Eating Fat Makes You Gain Weight'

Eating too much sugar is what causes our waistlines to grow. Fat does not make you fat. Fat is an appetite suppressant and we need it for survival. Healthiness of low-fat diets is one on the biggest myths in the health industry. Keeping fat out of your diet will lead you to be hungry and unsatisfied with your meals.

"The low-fat myth may have done more harm to the health of millions than any other dietary recommendation as the resulting low-fat craze led to increased consumption of trans-fats, which we now know increases your risk of obesity, diabetes and heart disease—the very health problems wrongfully attributed to saturated fats..."
-Dr.Mercola, *10 Lies and Misconceptions Spread By Mainstream Nutrition*

3. 'Artificial Sweeteners Are Safe Sugar-Replacements for Diabetics and Help Promote Safe Weight Loss'

"In 2005, data gathered from the 25-year long San Antonio Heart Study showed that drinking diet soft drinks increased the likelihood of serious weight gain, far more so than regular soda."

"3 On average, each diet soft drink the participants consumed per day increased their risk of becoming overweight by 65 percent within the next seven to eight years, and made them 41 percent more likely to become obese. There are several potential causes for this, including:

• Sweet taste alone appears to increase hunger, regardless of caloric content.

• Artificial sweeteners appear to simply perpetuate a craving for sweets, and overall sugar consumption is therefore not reduced—leading to further problems controlling your weight.4

• Artificial sweeteners may disrupt your body's natural ability to "count calories," as evidenced in studies such as this 2004 study at Purdue University,5 which found that rats fed artificially sweetened liquids ate more high-calorie food than rats fed high-caloric sweetened liquids.

There is also a large number of health dangers associated with artificial sweeteners and aspartame in particular. I've compiled an ever-growing list of studies pertaining to health problems associated with aspartame, which you can find here. If you're still on the fence, I highly recommend reviewing these studies for yourself so that you can make an educated decision."

-Dr.Mercola, *10 Lies and Misconceptions Spread By Mainstream Nutrition*

4. 'Your Body Can Not Tell the Difference Between Sugar and Fructose'

The public is being conditioned to believe that sugar and fructose are the "same." Fructose can and may be the main cause of why you have health and or weight problems. It is commonly overlooked and needs to be brought to people's attention that it is dangerous to health.

"Fructose is perhaps the greatest threat to your health. Mounting evidence testifies to the fact that excess fructose, primarily in the form of high fructose corn syrup (HFCS), is a primary factor causing not just obesity, but also chronic and lethal disease. In fact, I am convinced that fructose is one of the leading causes of a great deal of needless suffering from poor health and **premature death.**

Many conventional health 'experts,' contend that sugar and fructose in moderation is perfectly okay and part of a normal "healthy" diet, and the corn industry vehemently denies any evidence showing that fructose is metabolically more harmful than regular sugar (sucrose). This widespread denial and sweeping the evidence under the carpet poses a massive threat to your health, unless you do your own research."

-Dr.Mercola, *10 Lies and Misconceptions Spread By Mainstream Nutrition*

5. 'Soy Is A Health Food'

Soy products are promoted as being healthy but are far from it. Soy is marketed as "healthy" to get consumers to buy into the products and to feel better about what they are eating. It is used as cheap filler that takes the place of healthier ingredients. Soy is less damaging in fermented forms, but soy should not be a regular part of the diet in any form.

"Not only that, but more than 90 percent of American soy crops are genetically modified, which carries its own set of health risks.6 I am not opposed to all soy, however. Organic and, most importantly, properly fermented soy does have great health benefits. Examples of such healthful fermented soy products include tempeh, miso and natto. Here is a small sampling of the detrimental health effects linked to unfermented soy consumption."

-Dr.Mercola, *10 Lies and Misconceptions Spread By Mainstream Nutrition*

6. 'Eggs Are a Source of Unhealthy Cholesterol'

Eggs are a wonderful source of healthy fat and protein, are low carb and are filling. They are a food that has developed a bad reputation. The rumors pushed by the media about eggs are false. They are satisfying and can be a perfectly healthy, economical meal.

*"Eggs are probably one of the most demonized foods in the United States, mainly because of the misguided idea implied by the lipid hypothesis that eating egg yolk increases the cholesterol levels in your body. You can forget about such concerns, because contrary to popular belief, **eggs are one of the healthiest foods you can eat** and they do not have a detrimental impact on cholesterol levels. Numerous nutritional studies have dispelled the myth that you should avoid eating eggs, so this recommendation is really hanging on by a very bare thread…"*

-Dr.Mercola, **10 Lies and Misconceptions Spread By Mainstream Nutrition**

7. 'Whole Grains Are Good For Everyone'

"The use of whole-grains is an easy subject to get confused on especially for those who have a passion for nutrition, as for the longest time we were told the fiber in whole grains is highly beneficial. Unfortunately ALL grains, including whole-grain and organic varieties, can elevate your insulin levels, which can increase your risk of disease. They also contain gluten, which many are sensitive to, if not outright allergic. It has been my experience that more than 85 percent of Americans have trouble controlling their insulin levels -- especially those who have the following conditions:

- *Overweight*
- *Diabetes*
- *High blood pressure*
- *High cholesterol*
- *Protein metabolic types*

In addition, sub-clinical gluten intolerance is far more common than you might think, which can also wreak havoc with your health. As a general rule, I strongly recommend eliminating or at least restricting grains as well as sugars/fructose from your diet, especially if you have any of the above conditions that are related to insulin resistance. The higher your insulin levels and the more prominent your signs of insulin overload are, the more ambitious your grain elimination needs to be."

-Dr.Mercola, **10 Lies and Misconceptions Spread By Mainstream Nutrition**

8. 'Milk Does Your Body Good'

"Unfortunately, the myth that conventional pasteurized milk has health benefits is a persistent one, even though it's far from true. Conventional health agencies also refuse to address the real dangers of the growth hormones and antibiotics found inconventional[sic] milk. I do not recommend drinking pasteurized milk of any kind, including organic, because once milk has been pasteurized its physical structure is changed in a way that can actually cause allergies and immune problems.

Important enzymes like lactase are destroyed during the pasteurization process, which causes many people to not be able to digest milk. Additionally, vitamins (such as A, C, B6 and B12) are diminished and fragile milk proteins are radically transformed from health nurturing to unnatural amino acid configurations that can actually worsen your health. The eradication of beneficial bacteria through the pasteurization process also ends up promoting pathogens rather than protecting you from them.

The healthy alternative to pasteurized milk is **raw milk**, *which is an outstanding source of nutrients including beneficial bacteria such as lactobacillus acidophilus, vitamins and enzymes, and it is, in my estimation, one of the finest sources of calcium available. For more details please watch the* **interview I did with Mark McAfee**, *who is the owner of Organic Pastures, the largest organic dairy in the US [on www.mercola.com.]"*

-Dr.Mercola, *10 Lies and Misconceptions Spread By Mainstream Nutrition*

9. 'Genetically Engineered Foods Are Safe and Comparable to Conventional Foods'

"Make no mistake about it; genetically engineered (GE) foods may be one of the absolute most dangerous aspects of our food supply today. I strongly recommend avoiding ALL GE foods. Since over 90 percent of all corn grown in the US is GE corn, and over 95 percent all soy is GE soy, this means that virtually every processed food you encounter at your local supermarket that does not bear the 'USDA Organic' label likely contains one or more GE components."

-Dr.Mercola, *10 Lies and Misconceptions Spread By Mainstream Nutrition*

10."Lunch Meats Make For a Healthy, Nutritious Meal'

We all love a good sandwich and most people like lunch meats. If you do, you should be aware of some facts. You may be shocked about what you are eating on a daily basis. I hope this helps convince you to look for the healthier alternatives. So many people buy convenient foods, such as lunch meats and this can be so damaging to your health if you are not careful about what you are buying. Here is the expert's description.

"Lastly, processed meats, which includes everything from hot dogs, deli meats, bacon, and pepperoni are rarely thought of as strict no-no's, but they really should be, if you're concerned about your health. Virtually all processed meat products contain dangerous compounds that put them squarely on the list of foods to avoid or eliminate entirely. These compounds include:

• **Heterocyclic amines (HCAs)**: *a potent carcinogen, which is created when meat or fish is cooked at high temperatures.*

• *Sodium nitrite: a commonly used preservative and antimicrobial agent that also adds color and flavor to processed and cured meats.*

• *Polycyclic Aromatic Hydrocarbons (PAHs): Many processed meats are smoked as part of the curing process, which causes PAHs to form.*

• *Advanced Glycation End Products (AGEs): When food is cooked at high temperatures—including when it is pasteurized or sterilized—it increases the formation of AGEs in your food. AGEs build up in your body over time leading to oxidative stress, inflammation and an increased risk of heart disease, diabetes and kidney disease.*

This recommendation is backed up by a report commissioned by The World Cancer Research Fund8 (WCRF). The review, which evaluated the findings of more than 7,000 clinical studies, was funded by money raised from the general public, so the findings were not influenced by vested interests. It's also the biggest review of the evidence ever undertaken, and it confirms previous findings: Processed meats increase your risk of cancer, especially bowel cancer, and NO amount of processed meat is "safe." A previous analysis by the WCRF found that eating just one **sausage** *a day raises your risk of developing bowel cancer by 20 percent, and other studies have found that processed meats increase your risk of:*

• *Colon cancer by 50 percent*
• *Bladder cancer by 59 percent*
• *Stomach cancer by 38 percent*
• *Pancreatic cancer by 67 percent*

Processed meats may also increase your risk of diabetes by 50 percent, and lower your lung function and increase your risk of chronic obstructive pulmonary disease (COPD). If you absolutely want or need a hot dog or other processed meats once in awhile[sic], you can reduce your risk by:

• *Looking for "uncured" varieties that contain NO nitrates*

• *Choosing varieties that say 100% beef, 100% chicken, etc. This is the only way to know that the meat is from a single species and does not include byproducts (like chicken skin or chicken fat or other parts)*

• *Avoiding any meat that contains MSG, high-fructose corn syrup, preservatives, artificial flavor or artificial color Ideally, purchase sausages and other processed meats from a small, local farmer who can tell you exactly what's in their products. These are just some of the health myths and misconceptions out there. There are certainly many more. The ones listed above are some of the most important ones, in my view, simply because they're so widely misunderstood. They're also critical to get "right" if you want to protect your health, and the health of your loved ones. For more great advise, please review the two featured sources."*

-Dr.Mercola, **10 Lies and Misconceptions Spread By Mainstream Nutrition**

Dr. Mercola is a world-renowned, trusted natural health expert that has been discovering and spreading the truth about health for years. If more doctors cared about fixing the root of our health problems instead of covering up the symptoms with drugs, I believe we would all be better off. So many people rely on medications and pills to fix their problems. The goal is to remove one of the roots of the problem which is what you are putting into your body.

What Makes Me Fat But Not You? (& Vice Versa)

As you already know, there are a number of things that will add to your waistline. Food is the most obvious answer, but deeper down it is also stress, anxiety, how you think, and how much activity you get. We all have different bodies and we all react to everything differently. Some people are not allergic to peanuts, and others can't even smell it without having to go to the hospital. Isn't it amazing that the scent of something can do that to the human body? Imagine what eating large quantities of something that is damaging your body can do.

Gluttony is a word that is not very appealing. The definition of gluttony is "habitual greed or excess in eating." To be gluttonous is to be a greedy person. Those who are gluttonous about eating will tend to have a harder time losing weight. It seems like a basic concept, but so many people have trouble fixing the problem when gluttony is a factor.

You cannot blame the "type" of body you have for your weight problem. For instance, a lady I worked with when I was younger had a very hard time losing weight. She gained fat easily and seemed to put on the pounds simply by looking at a dessert. She's an extreme case, but there are others at the opposite end of the spectrum. There are people like my best friend who can eat anything and everything he wants without gaining an ounce. Everyone's body is different, but there should be no excuse when it comes to your health. There is a way to lose weight and to get healthy even if you feel you are the only one in the world that can't lose a pound.

First of all, with that attitude, you won't lose any weight. Second, you need to educate yourself on what makes you gain weight and how to lose weight in a healthy way; no fad diets or weight loss pills. Those are a fantasy! A pill will never do the job of helping you to lose weight. If you believe the fads the media is trying to sell you on, then I need you to think about this.

If there was really a quick fix weight-loss product available, don't you think everyone would be thin and in good shape? The truth is, taking care of yourself takes work and if you have done enough damage to yourself you can't expect to lose 50 pounds overnight. You're going to have to struggle through it.

Calorie Counting and Regulating Fat... Not What You Think

You probably read this chapter's title thinking, "Oh no! Anything but calorie counting!" Don't worry; you won't ever have to count a single calorie. You do not need to calorie count to lose weight. I have never a day in my life counted my calories and I probably never will. There is nothing wrong with counting your calories but calories are not what make you fat. It is the types of foods you are eating.

Overeating will catch up with anyone, but if you are just starting out and trying to lose weight, I wouldn't focus as much on counting your calories as I would focus on eliminating the excess carbohydrate, sugar and bad fat intake from your diet.

I can't tell you how many people I have heard say, "I can't eat that it has fat in it." I understand that to a degree. No one should be shoveling in French fries and pizza.

If you are serious about losing weight and about understanding what may be holding you back, you have to realize that you will have a difficult time losing weight without eating fat, and that you cannot survive without eating it.

Our bodies need fat- healthy fats from foods such as nuts, coconuts, olive oil, eggs, avocados and raw cheeses. Respectable doctors and health experts like Dr. Mercola and Dr. Ben Kim seem to agree.

Carbohydrates: Your Worst Enemy

Losing weight requires losing carbs in your diet. Carbohydrates add excess weight to your body. Sugar is one of the worst carbs you could be consuming. There are many foods loaded with carbs and sugar that are advertised as healthy when they are anything but healthy. Healthy carbs aren't hard to find. They are in foods such as fruits and vegetables. Those carbohydrates like those found in vegetables will keep you healthy in more ways than just losing weight.

It is the pasta, the pizza, the potatoes, the chips, the corn, the bread, and the sugary foods that are a big NO when losing weight. You will be amazed at how much weight you will lose in a week if you simply cut out the unhealthy excess carbs and stick to fruits, vegetables, meats, and healthy fats.

If are not willing to put the effort into your diet to make a change, you cannot complain about how you look and feel. When you cut the carbs and sugar from your everyday diet, your body won't be able to help but lose weight. You don't have to be hungry either. When you fill your meals with fruits, vegetables and grass-fed meats you will feel satisfied and you will not be hungry.

Your body needs fat to feel satisfied and full which is why it is so important you keep fat a part of your diet. It is the bad fats mixed with sugary carbohydrates like doughnuts, cookies and candy that will keep you farthest from your goal.

The best part about our bodies and this diet plan is that we get to continue to enjoy our favorite junk foods; they must simply be eaten in moderation. You have to earn the junk food. Just because you went to the gym and ran for a bit does not mean you get to reward yourself with a piece of cake afterwards. It is good that you are getting exercise if you do, but in another chapter we will touch on how weight loss starts with food.

You can exercise all day long, but if you are not fueling yourself properly your body will not run properly.

You can't let stress and comfort foods get in your way any longer. Strengthen your willpower and know that you have the answer- now you just need to take the steps and put what you know into action. When you feel like breaking, remember that every action has a consequence.

If that pleasure of a moment is more important to you than a lifetime of happiness and health, eat what you want instead of what you know you should. You have to discipline yourself. Your willpower will get stronger and the more results you see the more motivated you will become to keep going. Try it and see for yourself. You will not be disappointed.

Your Trusted Friends

How many friends do you have that you look up to and who are motivational? I hope the answer is 100% of them, but that is probably not likely. It is more likely that your friends have many of the same problems that you have. Maybe they are overweight and just can't seem to get on track or they are too busy to make a homemade meal, or they even believe the media's lies about food and what is healthy.

Generally, when someone is in your life that is at a higher level than you in whatever area it may be- health, financial, etc., you are put out of your comfort zone when you are around him or her.

I cannot even begin to tell you how good of a thing that can be for you. When someone puts you out of your comfort zone, you grow. The most successful people in this world surround themselves with like-minded individuals who they can learn from. They don't let their ego and being out of their comfort zone get in the way of what they are trying to succeed at in life.

Your friends should never keep you from being where you want to be in your life. If the people you surround yourself with bring you down and make you feel like what you are doing is "alright" just because they choose to live their lives that way does not mean it is okay.

If everyone in the office is going out to lunch every day, does that mean you have to do so? Instead of following the crowd, set a good example for everyone in the office and pack a homemade lunch and skip spending on a lunch that is probably adding to your problem. Are you worried about what others might think of you if you choose not to do what everyone else around you is doing?

The chances are that if you were to start a new healthy lifestyle you would be putting most of the people you are surrounded by out of their comfort zones. No one likes to feel like they are below someone else, or made to feel lazier than someone else.

Instead of feeling that way, learn from those around you who are doing the right thing and ask a lot of questions because this is the only way to make a change. Don't feel like you should follow the crowd just because it seems like the normal thing is to do.

Why Diets Don't Succeed

Diets don't succeed because when a person is trying to change the way he or she is living, it is not a diet change, it is a lifestyle change. A diet is used for short term fixes, when really it should be a lifestyle change for lasting results. Changes need to be things you can live with long-term, not things that you give up on after two weeks because they're too hard to live with. So note that when I say "diet" I really do mean a lifestyle change in your ways. We are in this for the long run, for your health and happiness long-term.

Diets also don't succeed because those selling diet products really don't want their products to work; they want you to keep buying. If these products worked, they would lose a customer. As I have said before, if there was some magic way to lose weight, everyone would be thin.

No one would feel the need to spend thousands of dollars on liposuction or weight loss products throughout their life. Weight loss should be done in a natural way. Your body reacts to food in specific ways, and as we discussed earlier you need to have the discipline to avoid all the bad food that is in production today. The vast array of items promoted as healthy never ceases to amaze me.

A healthy food should never have large amounts of sugar added to it like so many do. The healthiest food is the kind that has one ingredient- itself. If you want chicken, the only ingredient should be chicken. If you want some juice, the only ingredient should be that fruit from which the juice came. You then can season your food to taste good with spices and herbs. There are a million healthy ways to do this without adding preservatives and chemicals or dye to your food.

We have been conditioned to think otherwise. It is scary how many people do not realize that what they are putting in their bodies is killing them. If there is a list of 10 different strange ingredients on a label, you should not be putting this into your system.

You must be thinking ahead and be prepared when you are making a change in your lifestyle. If you plan on eating in a whole new way, be prepared by shopping ahead of time and sticking to your meal plans.

If you start a "diet" with no healthy food on hand to eat and a pantry full of junk, chances are you are going to cheat on it. Keep the junk out of your house. You will save money eating at home by not buying all the junk food you once did. You will be able to put more of your money toward healthy alternatives.

Elusive Benefits

Have you ever seen someone at the gym that spends hours sweating on the equipment day after day with no results? It can be a very frustrating, un-motivating thing to have happen. So many people spend too much time exercising and then they feel entitled to eat whatever they want when they get home. I give them credit for exercising, but you have to be focused on what you are eating even more so. Doing hours of cardio is not fun and is really not very effective if you are not cutting out the junk.

If you have to do hours of cardio to see results, this is a problem. You will most likely not stick to the new meal plan you have created for yourself and you will get burned out very quickly. If you are going to exercise, spend a good 20 to 30 minutes on a productive activity and then have something that compliments your workout instead of reverses it, such as a piece of fruit.

Not eating enough is not the answer to your weight loss problem, either. You will eventually break and binge on whatever you can get your hands on the fastest. Under-eating can be very dangerous to your health. When our bodies don't have food for long periods of time, we go into what is called survival mode and store fat instead of burn it. You will be stressed if you are hungry all the time and you will not have the energy to do everyday activities.

Time to Think Outside of the Box

When you keep doing the same thing over and over and don't see results, that is enough to make you go insane or just give up all together. Giving up certainly should not be an option when it comes to your health. Being overweight is not just something you should worry about for your physical appearance; it should be something you think about taking a toll on your overall health and your life span. Your actions will always catch up to you, good or bad. Maybe in high school you were thin and could eat whatever you wanted, but there is a point in time where you will have consequences for your actions.

Forgotten Food

Food is something that should be pure and safe to eat. Consumers tend to think nothing bad can happen to them until, well, something bad happens to them. No one is prepared for what comes with all the bad eating habits, lack of sleep, and stress. People can feel invincible until something happens to their bodies to make them take note.

It shouldn't take getting cancer or having diabetes to eat healthy. For some that is the case but it is never too late to begin anew. We take for granted the health we have and can be ignorant about changing our habits, even if it is life changing.

There used to be a time when food was truly natural and organic wasn't even a word thrown around because it was not needed. Food was simply organic-there were no chemicals and there were no preservatives, additives and addictive chemical ingredients. Today, organic food is not always accessible and often barely affordable. Also, our taste buds are not used to eating natural foods anymore, so healthy food has the bad reputation of being "bland."

Packaged and processed food is highly flavored and our tongues and taste buds don't even recognize good, plain, healthy food anymore.

When you change your eating habits and begin to eliminate the additives from your system, your taste buds will change. Whole food will taste good to you. You will not need to add sugar on top of the fruit you are eating because the natural sugars in it will be sweet enough to satisfy you.

It is sad that so much of our food has been tainted that we can't even enjoy a natural piece of fruit as it would taste right off of the tree.

There are places in the world that won't even allow many of the chemicals we add to our food to even be brought near the country. In Ecuador, their "organic" food is plentiful and inexpensive because it is all there is.

There are no pesticides used. In other places people can see the damage that adulterating food does to health and will not allow it in their homes or on their land. We have gone very astray in this country as far as food goes, and our health is paying the price. One in three people now has cancer and childhood obesity is at an all-time high. It is disturbing.

Teach Your Children Well

Maybe you have children, and maybe you don't. Either way, children are a reflection of their parents and how their parents behave. A child is normally born with a clean palate of taste buds. They have not yet been bombarded with junk food and chemicals that cause them to become addicted. I say yet because parents make the mistake of not introducing healthy foods early on in their child's life. If your children are given wholesome natural foods from the start, the chances are way higher of them not being picky about eating vegetables.

You are the parent, so you decide what they will be consuming. Teach your kids early before they have the chance to be brainwashed by the media that eating their vegetables is normal. Don't make a big deal out of something that shouldn't be a big deal to begin with. When you keep their taste buds pure, you will have a much easier time getting them to not only try new foods, but to love the healthy foods you give them.

My aunt has two children and she has done exactly this. Elise is 4 and Lance is 11. They are the only two kids I have ever met that simply eat whatever is put in front of them and do not complain. As a matter of fact, whenever we are at a family gathering or event, they order the most out of the ordinary food on the menu.

Things like squid and octopus, the things most kids would cry if you tried to get them to touch it, that's what they want. Spinach smoothies with only vegetables like carrots to give a touch of sweetness....others stand in awe as they ask for more.

They are both in great health and shape, their hair is shiny, they have perfect teeth and they glow. She keeps their bodies strong with healthy food. She takes the time to make homemade meals and taught them that it is a treat to eat candy, not an everyday event. Other parents are constantly impressed by how her kids eat and how healthy they are. Lance and Elise have been set up on a good path for a healthy life.

It is a wonderful thing that they will both be thanking my aunt for when they are older and have no health problems due to their eating habits. Her kids play outside in the summer and enjoy the fresh air and sunshine. They pick vegetables and herbs right from the garden and eat them. This seems so unusual in this day and age, but it should not be at all. Buying food in boxes should be unusual, but sadly has become the norm.

It is unfortunate how many children today are obese and would rather sit inside than to go out and play with a ball.

The schools are certainly no help promoting things like pizza and pretzels as "healthy." These kids are being brainwashed early on and if you have kids or plan on having them, the earlier you work with them on their habits the easier your life and their life will be. There is always time to help your child be the healthiest they can be.

Following Through

Results take effort and they take time. As I have said before, if you have done years of damage to your body you cannot expect to heal overnight. It is in our nature to be impatient and to not want to wait for things.

If you're going to take the time to plan new meals and to make the drastic change in your life of eating how you were meant to eat, then you have to have your mind set in the right place. You have to follow through with what you decide to do or you will keep putting off what you are capable of doing.

If you work hard every week, you will see results every week and you will keep yourself motivated. Nothing is more motivational than seeing results. Results will show you it is not impossible and you are another step closer to your goal. You must give yourself time to see the results. It will be well worth it.

We Believe Our Eyes and Ears Instead of Our Bodies

Our instinct should be to listen to our ears, eyes and all of our other senses. When we are being deceived by the media about our food this is not the case. The food that is good for us is not always regarded as it should be and the bad food is regarded to be all it is not.

They put pretty packaging, false advertising, fake coloring and addictive ingredients into many foods that are bought by families every day. Some people honestly believe the labels on the front of their child's juice box that says, "Made with real fruit juice!" I don't mean to be pessimistic, but do people read all the ingredients? Is fruit even near the first one? How much sugar is added to that healthy fruit juice box? How much dye is added to make the drink more appealing to the eye?

Again, it is your responsibility to know what you are putting into your body and to not rely on the enticing advertisement of a product to sway you into buying it. Listen to your body before your ears and eyes. Do you really feel good and energized after eating unhealthy food throughout your day? Do you feel good about your weight? Do you need change and do you need it now?

My mom always taught me to make a list for the store, stick to it and to come out with only the items on the list. There is a reason that stores put all that candy by the checkout lines, it is tempting you to buy as you stand and wait. Your children see it and ask for it. It was not placed there by accident; it was designed to be an impulse item you buy because you are caught up in having a moment of pleasure or by keeping your child happy.

No one wakes up and thinks, "Hey, I want to be fat when I am older or I want to be unhealthy today." We get caught up in buying what tastes good and enjoying comfort food and overeating and even drinking. Alcohol is one of the worst things you can consume if you want to lose any weight. It is one of the few things that builds fat and burns muscle at the same time. It is something to have in moderation, not every weekday night or every Friday and Saturday night.

It should be thought of as a treat and should be respected as that and that only. This goes for anything that can damage your health. If you are constantly eating chips as a snack and a carbohydrate-filled meal before bed, you can expect the results of your actions to be disappointing.

Re-engineering Your Mindset

Your mind is capable of so many things that it is what can make or destroy you. You have the power to have the willpower to make your goals a reality. You can wish for the weight to fall off and to continue feeling bad for yourself or you can realize that it is going to take work and dedication to be the person you want to be and that it is totally worth it. There is nothing more rewarding than improving your own self. You will set a good example for everyone around you and you will be respected. You are important and you deserve to live a happy, healthy life and you can start as soon as now.

Constantly thinking about what you want to do will not get you there. You have to take the actions and do it. This is not only in respect to weight loss; it applies to any area of your life you want to improve.

We take such advantage of the way we eat. Food is something that was meant for survival in the early stages of human existence. Today, it is used for pleasure. I love food as much as the next person. I love cooking and making new recipes and eating junk food, too! Does this mean I take advantage of what is being sold to me?

Definitely not, because I understand that eating something like cheesecake is a reward for a week of eating healthy. I have no guilt when I eat the things I love when it is in moderation. Moderation is not every night of the week, or even 5, it is maybe one day a week. If you eat no carbs, no sugar and no processed food for 6 days and then splurge on a cheat meal maybe on a Saturday night, you will be losing weight and regaining your health in no time.

Even when I make a dessert, I use unbleached, unbromated flour, free range eggs and other pure ingredients. Desserts don't have to be loaded with bad ingredients to be enjoyable. There are so many healthy alternatives to harmful foods that you can easily learn to make and enjoy. I have invested the time in myself to learn to cook and bake a little so that I can prepare my own food because my health comes before everything else.

Your health is the most important part of your life. Without your health, you cannot live.

I put together this collection of food knowledge in order to help you protect your family, your loved ones, and, most importantly, yourself. It's not very often you find someone in this world who treats your health as delicately as you do. Please, take advantage of the opportunity. I want you to have a long, fulfilling, and healthy life.

I see it like this:

"If I don't have my health, I have nothing."
-Alexandra Kastor

Wait Before You Go!

As a special thanks to you, our reader, please accept this FREE gift!

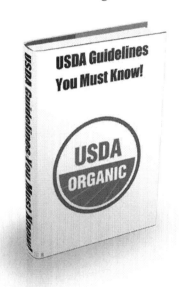

Purchasing this book may have been the first step of your journey to a better life. As a thank you for your purchase, and to help you on this journey, I would like to provide to you a **USDA Organic Guidelines Report Absolutely FREE.**

Download at:

alexandsteven.com/signups/saltsugarfat

More by This Bestselling Author!

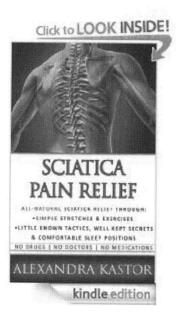

Sciatica Pain Relief (Our Bestseller!)

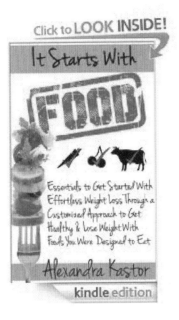

It Starts With Food (Our Newest Addition!)

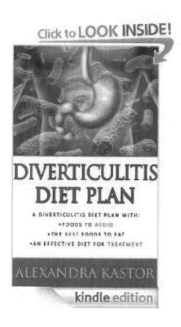

Diverticulitis Diet Plan (Includes Foods to Avoid and Eat!)

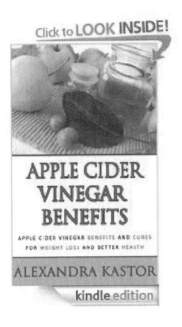

Apple Cider Vinegar Benefits (Over 1,000 Copies Sold!)

Resources

- http://www.mediaite.com/online/poll-americans-confidence-in-television-media-falls-to-all-time-low/
- http://www.amazon.com/gp/product/B009K54F48/ref=as_li_ss_tl?ie=UTF8&camp=1789&creative=390957&creativeASIN=B009K54F48&linkCode=as2&tag=tech0271-20
- http://www.marketplace.org/topics/life/big-book/processed-foods-make-70-percent-us-diet
- http://www.elephantjournal.com/2013/04/sneaky-names-for-msg-check-your-labels/
- http://aspartame.mercola.com/
- http://articles.mercola.com/sites/articles/archive/2009/10/13/artificial-sweeteners-more-dangerous-than-you-ever-imagined.aspx
- http://articles.mercola.com/sites/articles/archive/2003/07/19/trans-fat-part-three.aspx
- http://www.huffingtonpost.com/2012/05/11/fruit-roll-ups-lawsuit_n_1509650.html
- http://www.huffingtonpost.com/2013/03/08/artificial-food-dye-kraft-macaroni-and-cheese_n_2837205.html
- http://articles.mercola.com/sites/articles/archive/2013/02/25/mainstream-nutrition-biggest-lies.aspx
- http://articles.mercola.com/sites/articles/archive/2010/07/31/aspartame-update.aspx

- http://articles.mercola.com/sites/articles/archive/2009/11/24/Spoonful-Of-Sugar-Makes-The-Worms-Life-Span-Go-Down.aspx
- http://articles.mercola.com/sites/articles/archive/2010/05/01/mark-mcafee-interview.aspx
- http://articles.mercola.com/sites/articles/archive/2008/06/19/can-grilling-meat-cause-cancer.aspx
- http://articles.mercola.com/sites/articles/archive/2008/04/17/eating-just-one-sausage-a-day-raises-your-cancer-risk-by-20-percent.aspx
- http://articles.mercola.com/sites/articles/archive/2011/09/01/enjoy-saturated-fats-theyre-good-for-you.aspx
- http://drbenkim.com/articles-fat.html

©2013, Alexandra Kastor & Affiliates
ISBN-13: **978-0615880730**
ISBN-10: **0615880738**
(A&S Publishing)

29078505R00040

Made in the USA
Lexington, KY
12 January 2014